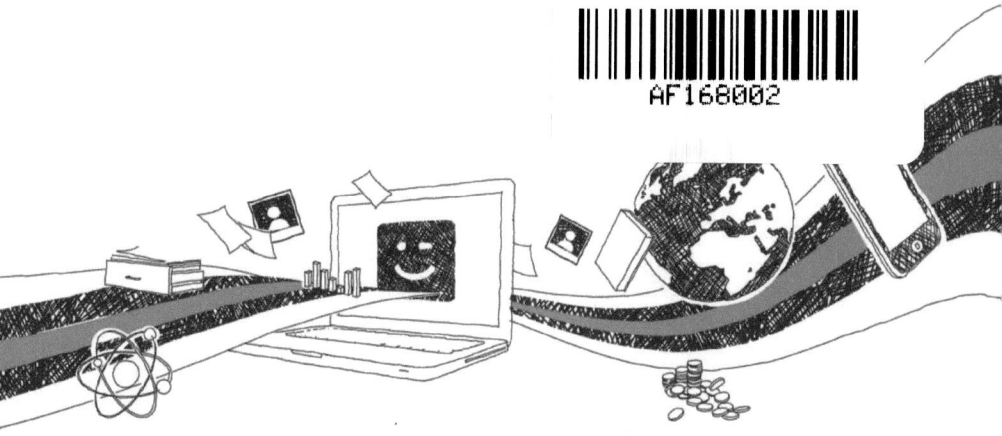
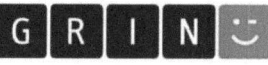

The Current Relevance of Tuberculosis in Germany

Ulrich Schmitz

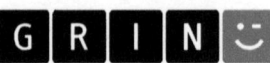

Bibliographic information published by the German National Library:

The German National Library lists this publication in the National Bibliography; detailed bibliographic data are available on the Internet at http://dnb.dnb.de.

ISBN: 9783346195555
This book is also available as an ebook.

Print and binding: Books on Demand GmbH, Norderstedt, Germany
Printed on acid-free paper from responsible sources.

The present work has been carefully prepared. Nevertheless, authors and publishers do not incur liability for the correctness of information, notes, links and advice as well as any printing errors.

GRIN web shop: https://grin.extdb.e-fellows.net/document/906536

INCORPORATING GLOBAL HEALTHCARE INTO THE ORGANISATION

Tuberculosis in Germany Today

Ulrich Schmitz
Manchester Metropolitan University

Content

Introduction

This essay aims to highlight the present relevancy of Tuberculosis in Germany. The disease and its global threat will be discussed as well as the response of the government to prevent spread into Germany. Finally, implications for dental practices will be mentioned.

The Importance of Tuberculosis Today

TB played a big role in history. So, the "big white plague" remains about 200 years until 1900 and killed more than 1 billion people in Europe (Kerksiek, 2009). The disease influenced art and music of those times, as the health of famous people like Matthias Claudius, Friedrich Schiller, Carl Maria von Weber, and Frederic Chopin was affected, too.

Today, citizens of developed countries nearly don't know even the name "Tuberculosis". This lack of knowledge doesn't stop in front of the healthcare system; TB seems to be just a historical note.

Till the year 2015 Tuberculosis was said to be defeated in Germany. Only 5,865 new infections, less than 0.05 % of cases all over the world, were counted at the time (Hillienhof, 2016).

In contrast to that situation, worldwide the disease spread enormously, so today it is still one of the top 10 causes of death (WHO, 2018).

Top causes of death worldwide in 2016.[a,b]
Deaths from TB among HIV-positive people are shown in grey.

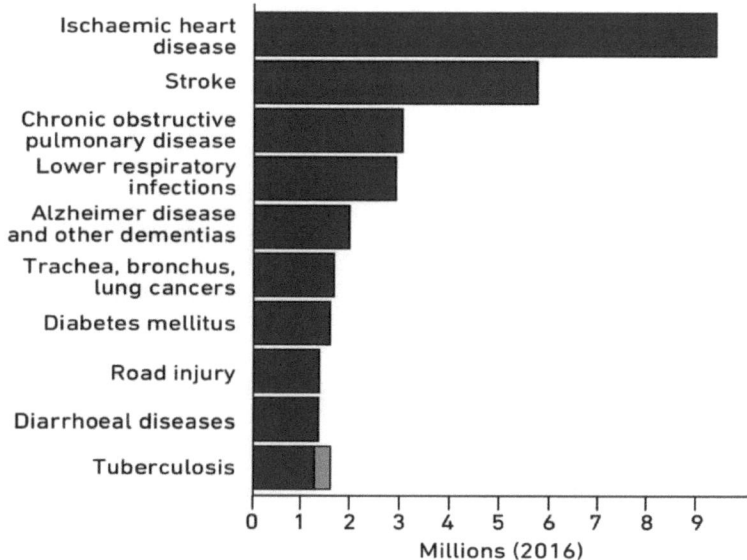

[a] This is the latest year for which estimates for all causes are currently available. See WHO estimates, available at http://apps.who.int/gho/portal/uhc-fp-cabinet-wrapper-v2.jsp?id=1020201 (accessed 15 August 2018).
[b] Deaths from TB among HIV-positive people are officially classified as deaths caused by HIV/AIDS in the International classification of diseases.

Figure 1: Causes of Death in 2016 (WHO, 2018)

Current Situation in Germany

Nevertheless, 2015 may be recognised as a turning point in Germany, as there were clearly

lower infections in 2013 (4,325 cases) and 2014 (4,533 cases).

The important finding to consider is the distribution of the cases in 2015:

1,255 cases, about 22 %, were diagnosed in asylum seekers (Hillienhof, 2016).

Beginning in 2015 with a peak in autumn 2015 more than 1 million refugees and migrants

entered Germany. Most of them arrived from Syria (caused by the civil war), Iraq, Afghanistan,

Balkan States, and several states in Africa. These are all home countries with significant higher

TB incidence rates, as the WHO-map shows.

Estimated TB incidence rates, 2015

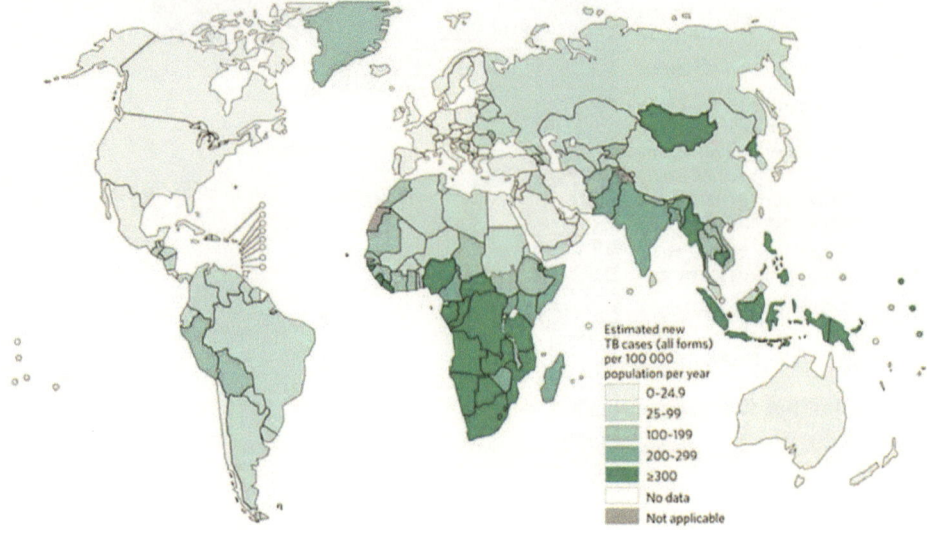

(WHO / Global tuberculosis report 2016)

Figure 2: Estimated TB incidence rates, 2015

This enormous number of people led to the highest number of asylum applications ever,

476,649 after 273,815 in 2014 (BMI-Press, 2016). In 2016 there was another extreme growth

up to 745,545.

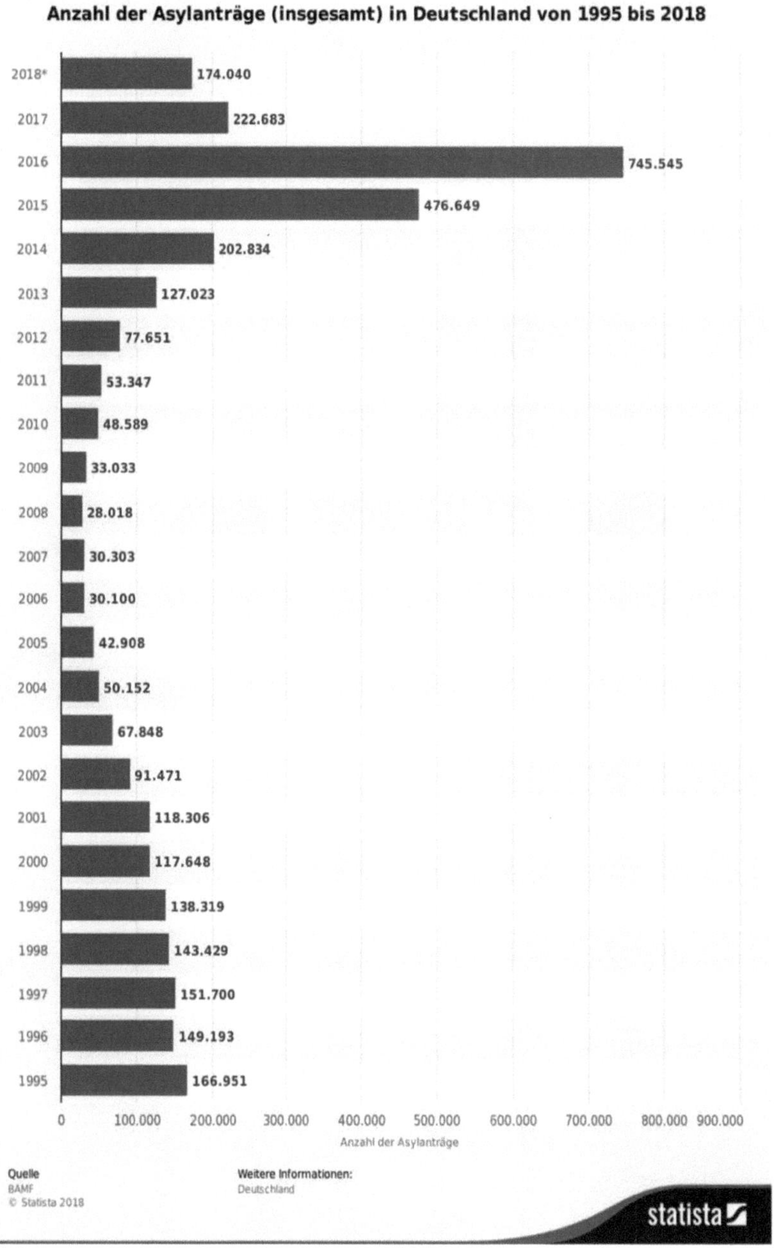

Anzahl der Asylanträge (insgesamt) in Deutschland von 1995 bis 2018

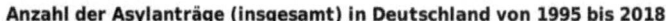

Jahr	Anzahl
2018*	174.040
2017	222.683
2016	745.545
2015	476.649
2014	202.834
2013	127.023
2012	77.651
2011	53.347
2010	48.589
2009	33.033
2008	28.018
2007	30.303
2006	30.100
2005	42.908
2004	50.152
2003	67.848
2002	91.471
2001	118.306
2000	117.648
1999	138.319
1998	143.429
1997	151.700
1996	149.193
1995	166.951

0   100.000   200.000   300.000   400.000   500.000   600.000   700.000   800.000 900.000

Anzahl der Asylanträge

Quelle
BAMF
© Statista 2018

Weitere Informationen:
Deutschland

statista

Figure 3: Number of asylum applications (in total) in Germany from 1995 to 2018
Statista, 2018

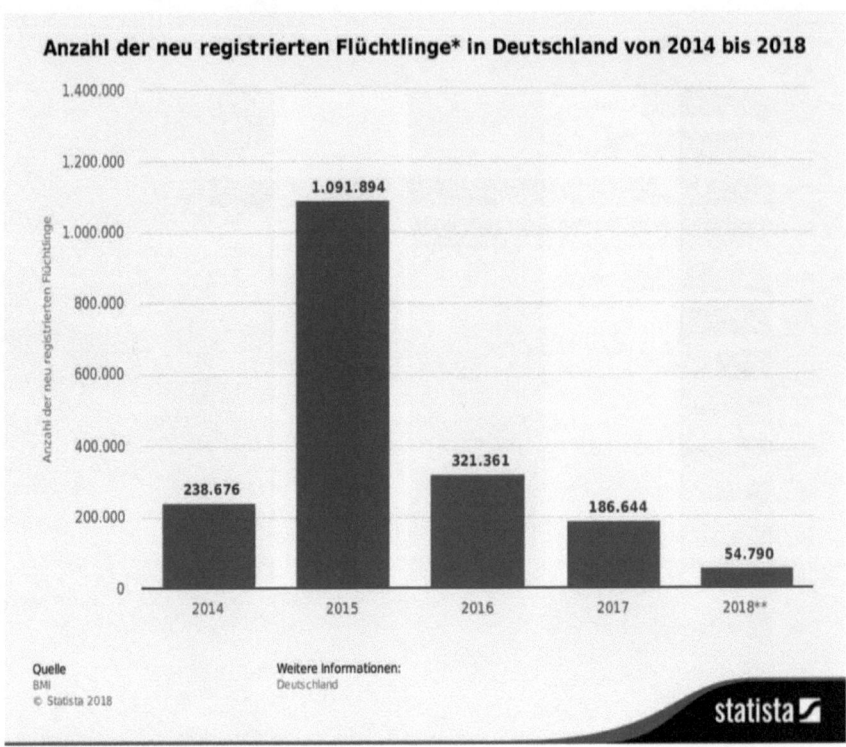

Figure 4: Number of newly registered refugees in Germany from 2014 to 2018, (Statista, 2018)

The assimilation of all those people challenges society and not everyone welcomes these new citizens. Especially right-wing politicians try to create a climate of fear. A field they like to use is the assumed danger of contamination with fatal diseases imported by refugees.

The one, mostly mentioned in this context by politicians and media, is **Tuberculosis**.

An objective, scientific view will help to decide, if there is a real and growing danger of Tuberculosis in Germany today.

Tuberculosis and its Nature of Threat

The Disease

As a foundation the main characteristics and communication paths of the disease are introduced. The knowledge of these facts is necessary to understand the potential danger and find an appropriate way for protection.

TB is caused by the Mycobacterium tuberculosis (MTB), first discovered by Robert Koch, a German physician and microbiologist in 1882. Bacteria are spread via droplet infection from sufferers through coughing, sneezing, spitting, or even speaking and singing.

Two forms of the disease have to be distinguished:

- **Latent TB**, which shows no clinical symptoms.

    More than a quarter of the world's population (> 2 Billion) is infected with MTB, which is ubiquitous since ancient times (Adams and Woelk, 2014). These otherwise healthy persons are not thought to be contagious (Kumar et al., 2007), but even though MTB grows very slowly over a lifetime - depending on the immune system - about 10 % of them develop the active form (Sundareshan and Evans, 2009).

    Risk factors which increase the likelihood of progression are:

    - Co-diseases: Diabetes mellitus (Restrepo, 2007), Renal Failures (Adams and Woelk, 2014)

    - Poor Nutrition and Overcrowding (Poverty!) (Lawn and Zumla, 2011)

    - Smoking (van Zyl Smit et al., 2010)

    - Immune Suppression (medications like Steroids and Infliximab) (Lawn and Zumla, 2011)

    - HIV Infection – the most important co-factor (WHO, 2018)

- **Active TB**, which shows a death rate of about 45 % without proper treatment (WHO, 2018).

Typical clinical symptoms are cough with blood-containing sputum due to an affected lung, fever, night sweats, and excessive weight loss.

These patients may transmit MTB from the beginning of the involvement of the lungs. This **pulmonary form** makes up about 90 % of active cases (Behera, 2010). If the bacilli break outside the lung every organ may be infected (Crowley, 2010). A severe form of the **extrapulmonary TB** with many foci is known as **Miliary TB**, which leads to death in about 30 % though adequate treatment is applied (Jacob et al., 2009).

The Potential Threat

According to the WHO (2018), Tuberculosis is the number one infectious cause of death worldwide. It occurs all over the world but there are high burden countries. Several programs are set up to build a TB-free world with the goal of ending the epidemic by 2030 (Lancet Commission, 2018). Also, "a 2035 target of 95 % reduction in deaths and a 90 % decline in TB incidence – similar to current levels in low TB incidence countries today" (WHO, 2014) is defined.

Though an action framework for low-incidence countries exists since 2014 (Fiebig et al., 2015), it seems, as if the maintenance of the current state in developed countries is neglected. Situations may change and a never completely eradicated disease will adapt and spread again.

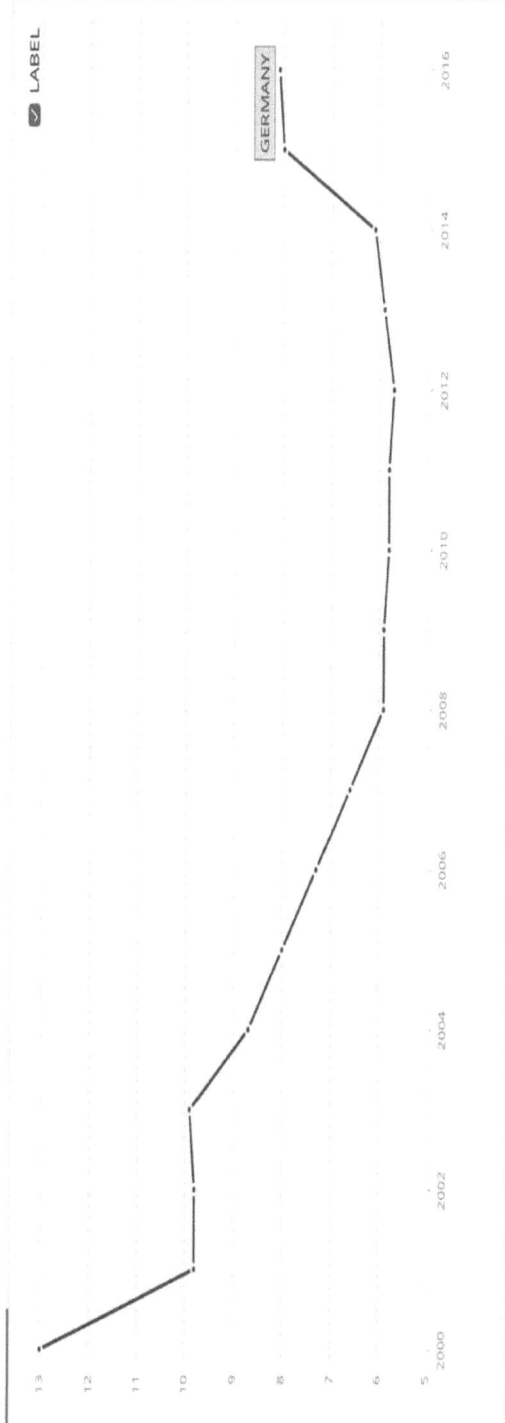

Figure 5: Incidence of TB in Germany (The World Bank, 2018)

9

The main unforeseen new challenges in controlling TB over the last decades are:

- Occurrence of HIV

  This viral disease was recognised for the first time in 1981. The infection damages the immune system and exhausts the response. That makes HIV a perfect driver of the TB epidemic (Adams and Woelk, 2014). The WHO (2018) reports a 20 to 30 times higher likelihood of developing an active TB for HIV-patients. The "partnership" of an ancient disease with an emerging one even strengthens their fatal power. Currently, TB is the leading cause of mortality among HIV patients.

- Drug-Resistance

  During the 1990s resistance to first-line drugs (isoniazid and rifampin) became a worldwide threat (CDC, 2006). Second-line drugs (SLDs) where required, which were less effective, more toxic and costlier (CDC, 2006). Already at that time about 2 % XDR (extensively drug-resistant) cases were found. Nearly no SLD was able to cure that TB. Today drug resistance is detected using special laboratory tests to speed up and improve outcomes (WHO, 2018).

- Failure of Vaccine

  Till today only one vaccine is approved worldwide, the nearly 100-year-old BCG-Vaccine for children. As it doesn't protect against the most common form, the pulmonary type of young adults, in Germany no newborn baby has vaccinated anymore (STIKO [Ständige Impfkommission/Permanent Vaccination Commission], RKI, 2018). The development of a new vaccine wouldn't only be helpful in the containment of the disease, but it could be the most important weapon against resistant MTB (Kaufmann and Schrager, 2016).

- Migration, Tourism

  These are the most current topics today. As TB cannot be seen in a person's face and

  detection of MTB will take at least several hours with the use of a laboratory, which is

  costly, it is not possible to close entry points and borders of a country.

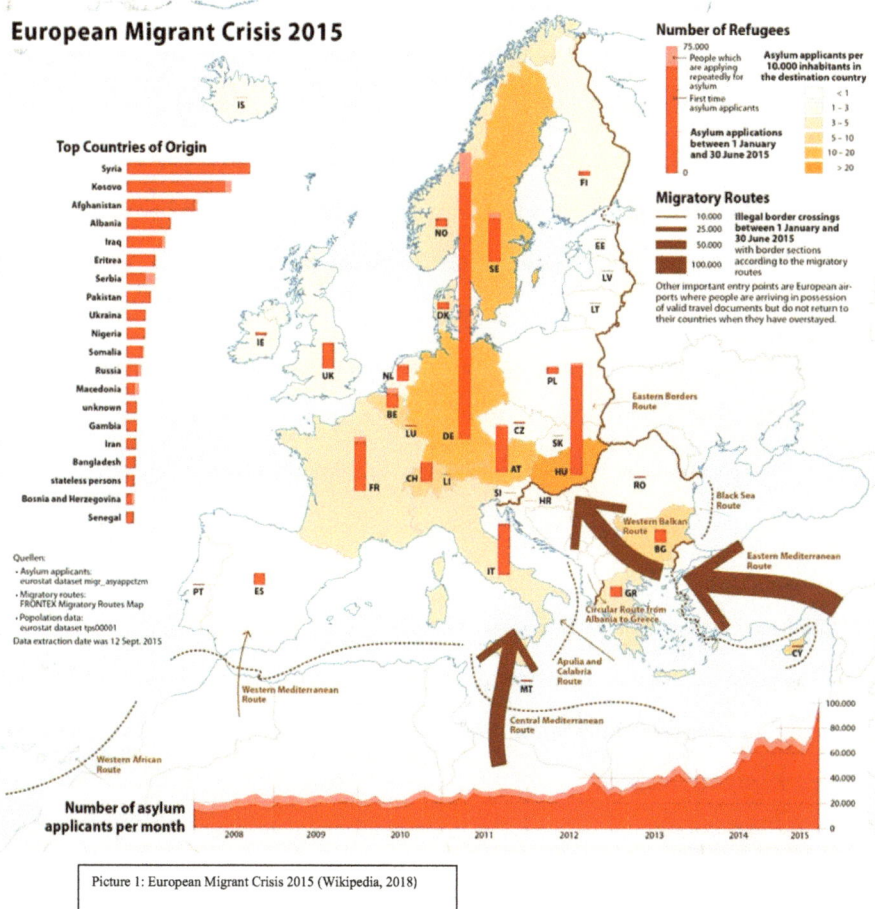

Three different forms of entering must be distinguished:

1. Citizens of the country come back from a journey to a high-burden part of the world

   infected with TB.

   Only a very small number of persons is concerned, who doesn't represent a danger

   for a nation's health status.

11

2. Infected people come to Germany to get medical aid. As long as those patients have appointments with specialised clinics and are willing to pay for their treatment, that won't cause any problems. But there could be patients without any appointments or money, who may spread TB.

3. Difficult to control is the number of refugees and migrants arriving from high-burden countries. Many of them don't have any passports and won't live in free collective living quarters, where a medical check-up is mandatory. A considerable number enters Germany without any (health) control. Reliable figures aren't published, so this represents a playground especially for right-wing politicians and the yellow press. Using numbers investigated by a typically trustworthy TV-report (Spiegel-TV, 2015) there could be about 8,000 – 10,000 migrants with serious TB, who entered Germany in 2015. That number doesn't seem to be a danger for the population but compared with numbers of around 5,000 cases in the years till 2014 that is a real challenge for the healthcare system.

Challenges for the German Healthcare System

To be successful in a fight against an epidemic infection several requirements have to be met locally. They represent different challenges for members of the healthcare system and not all are currently under control.

1. The disease and its characteristics should be well-known by healthcare staff.

   Basics about TB are taught at universities and healthcare schools. As it seemed to be defeated in Germany till 2014 there was no particular emphasis put on knowledge sharing. It will take several years to implement an updated syllabus. The release of a "S2k-Guideline", which summarises current knowledge about diagnosis and therapy (Schaberg et al., 2017), marks a first step in the right direction.

2. A patient with symptoms must be recognised and examined.

Usually, a patient sees her/his family doctor before she/he is referred to a specialist or hospital.

A dissertation (Broennecke, 2014) found a significant lack of knowledge among primary care physicians. Just one TB-patient to 14 physicians is shown statistically in 2009. That may be a reason for lost knowledge. Especially questions about obligations to notify authorities and drug resistance weren't answered well. As a result, diagnosis and start of an adequate therapy may be retarded.

A small number of physicians, who had taken extra continuing education (CME) in TB over the last three years, presented significantly advanced knowledge.

The offer of free or at least cheap CME about TB for all members of the healthcare system, who may get in touch with the disease, would be helpful to prevent a resurgence of TB even in low-incidence countries. If it would be possible to create a feeling of urgency, that may be an easy way to get a great number of physicians updated with the necessary knowledge.

3. It is required that persons feeling ill visit a practice or a hospital or be detected actively. In countries like Germany TB concentrates in certain at-risk groups like homeless people, people living with HIV, people with harmful alcohol or drug use, and migrants (WHO, 2018). All these people normally don't see any healthcare worker regularly, mostly because they have neither medical insurance nor own money to pay for. Other barriers may be culture, missing language skills, or unfamiliarity to the insurance and healthcare system.

Assuming only a part of sick persons will visit a practice, this passive detection should be extended by an active search. Specially educated healthcare workers should see those members of at-risk groups regularly.

Current migration poses a special issue. In addition to legal migrants and refugees, who may be examined at the entry points, there is a high number of illegal migrants (Aust

13

and Bewarder about GASIM report, 2017). It is impossible to get an overview of the state of health of those people, which may cause some uncertainties.

4. Necessary drugs and clinic spaces for treatment must be available.

In Germany, all drugs for a therapy of the uncomplicated TB and sufficient medications for therapy of MDR – or XDR-TB are available (Diel, 2014). Problems may occur in another field. Hospitals won't be able to offer the needed spaces and the medical staff at once to treat the increasing number of patients. It shouldn't be forgotten, that patients with active forms of TB must be isolated.

5. The treatment must be payable by healthcare insurances or patients.

Costs of therapy are covered by insurances. At first sight, that seems to be a positive message, but it only applies to direct medical costs, which include:

- Laboratory
- Outpatient treatment
- Inpatient care
- medication

There are more costs to consider.

o The patient needs time for recovery and rehabilitation, money for aids and appliances, and has to live with a reduced or missing income.

o The community is burdened with the loss of productivity, Germany loses about 50 Million € each year (Kaufmann and Schrager, 2016).

However, just the primary medical costs add up to large amounts (Diel et al., 2012):

- One TB patient = 7,500 €
- One MDR-TB patient = 52,300 €
- Overall TB-costs in Germany 2012 = 35 Million €

According to the rising number of patients, this amount will grow in the following years, though figures like 200,000 € per patient, as used in the press in 2015, seem to be exaggerated.

Nevertheless, it is a significant charge for insurance companies, especially if they are responsible for people, who didn't pay in any dues.

6. Guidelines of treatment must be followed by the patient (and known by therapists).

The past showed the importance of an exact following of all treatment guidelines. Non-compliance of patients or lack of knowledge of physicians led to drug resistances of MTB (WHO, 2018). As mentioned above continuing education may solve the issue on the side of healthcare providers, on the other side patients must be educated, too and monitored to avoid inappropriate handling of the medication.

The Response of the Government

The WHO published guidelines for low-incidence countries in 2014. Eight bullet points summarise recommendations on how to reach the goal of "End TB" (Appendix 1). Pre-elimination (incidence of 1/100,000) should be achieved by 2035, elimination (1/1,000,000) by 2050. Unfortunately, the downward trend in Germany changed in 2012 (Fiebig et al., 2015), even before the start of the refugee crisis in Europe.

There are different ways to explain the rise of cases:

- Real increase in cases
- Increased active detecting and reporting, which plays a major role since 2015, because migrants, who enter first-admission facilities, are checked actively.
- Artefacts may occur by double registration after movements of refugees or migrants within Germany.

So, it seems to be impossible to get a correct picture from available numbers, estimations may be influenced by interested parties.

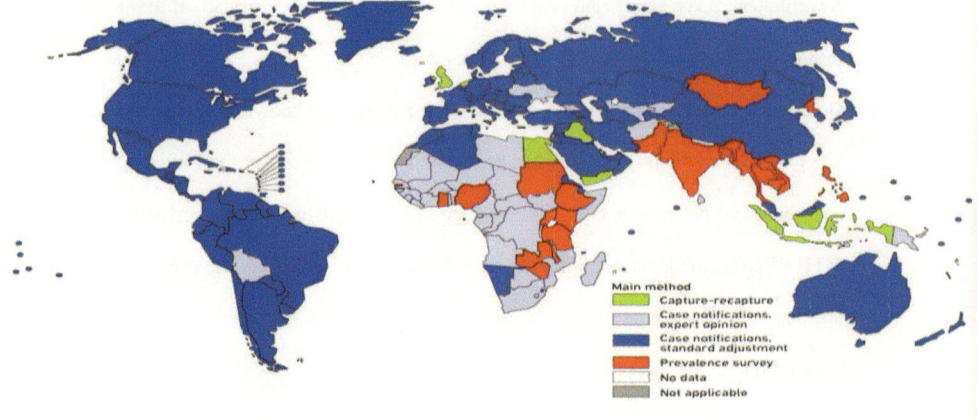

Fig. 6: Main Methods (WHO, 2018)

The Approach in Germany

Since 1998 the BCG vaccination is not recommended by STIKO anymore due to low protective effects (50 – 80%) and low risks of infection according to WHO recommendations (RKI, 2015). No vaccines are licensed in Germany. Therefore, different ways of control have to be established.

Today, physicians are obligated to report condition and death on TB, as well as refusal or discontinuation of TB treatment (RKI, 2013) to local authorities. The government agency and research institute to monitor and prevent public health in Germany, which collects these data, is named Robert Koch Institute (RKI) in honour of the discoverer of MTB.

At the institute, the information will be analysed and further steps to examine people from the environment of reported patients will be initiated.

The nature of the disease represents a specific challenge to detect especially the latent form. As a common screening test the Mendel-Mantoux-Test is used, where antigens of MTB are injected into the skin of the lower arm. More specific is a laboratory-based Interferon-Gamma-

Release Assay. Costs of about 100 – 150 € per modern test are mostly charged to the statutory health insurance.

The numbers indicate that not only treatment costs, but also detection costs of TB represent an important factor, which needs policy-based assistance.

The Response to the "Refugee Crisis"

Caused by the number of migrants and refugees pros and cons of different ways of detecting TB have to be evaluated. As a representative of the government guidelines released by the RKI needs to comply like laws. In 2015 two statements were published:

1. Thorax-Röntgenuntersuchungen bei Asylsuchenden gemäß § 36 Absatz 4 IfSG (05.10.2015) (Thorax-x-ray examinations among asylum seekers)

   People, older than 15 years, have to present a medical certificate before joining a shared saccommodation by law. The x-ray is mandatory. Though it is difficult and expensive to take x-rays of so many people, the RKI didn't recommend any other examination of equal value.

2. Untersuchung auf Tuberkulose bei asylsuchenden Kinder und Jugendlichen < 15 Jahre (16.12.2015) (TB-examination among young asylum seekers < 15 years)

   As the attendance at school and kindergarten is aimed as soon as possible the risk of transmission has to be eliminated to protect the general population. To avoid expensive examinations of surrounding people an IGRA for all children < 15 years is recommended. Positive tested persons need an x-ray as a second step.

The implementation of those measures requires high effort in time, money, and working capacity. But it will be worth in different ways. On the one hand, it is easier and cheaper to carry out careful detection than paying for illness and lost confidence. On the other hand, it should be remembered that nearly all of the refugees really need help.

Health is no topic for political wing infights, only joint efforts not only of one country but of all nations of the world will be strong enough to win against the "new global TB" and to fulfil the WHO strategy.

Conclusion

As outlined above the main challenges to succeed in fighting against a spread of TB are:

- Raising the awareness of this ancient disease among the national population
- Obligatory (Continuing) Education for healthcare workers, especially for those, who may be in first contact with migrants and refugees
- Active searching and reporting of "positive" cases
- Availability of funds for sufficient local examinations and treatment of entering people
- Support for research and development to find new drugs and vaccines globally

All these measures don't work alone, there should be a masterplan to protect the national population managed by the government and the RKI. But no one can be identified. So state-of-the-art examinations of asylum seekers are mandated, but performance isn't guaranteed. No new funds are established, a big part of the costs burdens the compulsory health insurances.

Latest RKI publication states the German population still as not vulnerable, as cases are declining in 2017 to 5486 with an incidence of 6.7 (RKI, 2018). The higher level in total should relate to active case finding for refugees.

The termination of a monthly report about notifiable infectious diseases in asylum seekers in December 2017 (RKI, 2018) fits into that picture.

Food for thought should be some different facts:

- TB incidence in German citizens 2.2 vs. 40.6 in foreign nationals residing in Germany (RKI, 2018)

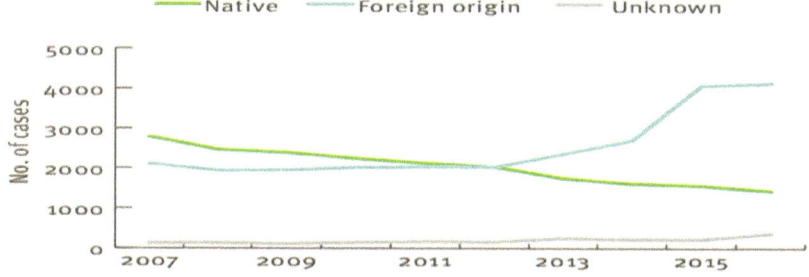

Tuberculosis cases by geographical origin, 2007–2016

— Native — Foreign origin — Unknown

- MDR-TB raised again in 2017 up to 3.0 %

  German citizens 1.0 % vs. 19.3 % nationals of the former Soviet Union residing in Germany (RKI, 2018)

- Germany shows the highest increase in TB notification rate of only 6 out of 35 European countries with incidences < 20 between 2012 and 2016 (ECDC, 2018).

- All statistics and calculations are based on reported cases. An unknown number of unreported cases may increase official figures.

It seems as if the potential threat of TB, especially the XDR-TB, isn't taken seriously by the government. Responsible authorities rely on official incidences, which still look well compared to most of the other countries worldwide. But the development of the situation in the world teaches that there are no borders for MTB. Its power grows, as currently, no drugs to defeat XDR-TB are available. Though it may be politically charged to provide funds for the extinction of a repressed ancient disease, this would be necessary to protect citizens in the future. Not only examinations of entering people must be paid but supporting international research about new vaccines to tackle the disease at its source promises sustained success.

Implications for a Dental Practice

The dental staff works at the interface of contagion, the mouth. This is a place with many other risks of infection. Common colds and flu are most known. Therefore, no additional safety steps must be taken, but present measures must be followed carefully. To ensure it, all staff members should be instructed about the transmission of TB and its current danger. To protect staff and patients the RKI guidelines about hygiene (DAHZ, 2018) must be followed meticulously.

It should be kept in mind that TB-patients may visit every practice today, not only specialist facilities, as it was in the years before 2015.

Abbreviations

BCG	Bacillus Calmette-Guérin
(*US*)CDC	Centers for Disease Control and Prevention
CME	Continuing Medical Education
ECDC	European Centre for Disease Prevention and Control
GASIM	Gemeinsames Analyse- und Strategiezentrum illegale Migration (Common Assay- and Strategy-centre illegal Migration)
HIV	Human Immunodeficiency Virus
IGRA	Interferon-Gamma-Release Assay
LTBI	Latent Tuberculosis Infection
MDR	Multi drug-resistant
MTB	Mycobacterium tuberculosis
RKI	Robert Koch Institute
SLD	Second-Line Drug
STIKO	Ständige Impfkommission (Permanent Vaccination Commission)
TB	Tuberculosis
WHO	World Health Organization
XDR	Extensively drug-resistant

Appendix 1

Eight Priority Actions (WHO, 2014)

1. Ensure political commitment, funding and stewardship for planning and essential services of high quality.

2. Address the most vulnerable and hard-to-reach groups.

3. Address special needs of migrants and cross-border issues.

4. Undertake screening for active TB and LTBI in TB contacts and selected high-risk groups, and provide appropriate treatment.

5. Optimize the prevention and care of drug-resistant TB.

6. Ensure continued surveillance, programme monitoring and evaluation and case-based data management.

7. Invest in research and new tools.

8. Support global TB prevention, care and control.

References

Adams, L. and Woelk, G. (2014) Tuberculosis and HIV/AIDS, editors Markle, W.H., Fisher, M.A., Smego, R.A. Understanding Global Health, McGraw-Hill: New York

Aust, S. and Bewarder, M. (2017) Anstieg illegaler Migration in der zweiten Jahreshälfte, Die Welt, accessed from: https://www.welt.de/167409477

Behera, D. (2010) Textbook of Pulmonary Medicine (2nd ed.). New Delhi: Jaypee Brothers Medical Publishers. p. 457. ISBN 978-81-8448-749-7.

BMI-Press (2016) 2015: Mehr Asylanträge in Deutschland als jemals zuvor, accessed from: https://www.bmi.bund.de/SharedDocs/pressemitteilungen/DE/2016/01/asylantraege-dezember-2015.html

Brönnecke, M. (2014) Kenntnisstand zur Tuberkulose unter hausärztlich tätigen Ärztinnen und Ärzten in Deutschland, Med. Diss. Charité – Universitätsmedizin Berlin

CDC (2006) Emergence of Mycobacterium tuberculosis with Extensive Resistance to Second-Line Drugs – Worldwide, 2000-2004, MMWR Weekly 55 (11), pp 301-305

DAHZ (2018) Hygieneleitfaden, 12. Ausgabe

Diel, R., Rutz, S., Castell, S., Schaberg, T. (2012) Tuberculosis: Cost of illness in Germany, Eur Resp J 20132(40), pp 143-151

Diel, R. (2014) Behandlungskosten für Tuberkulose und MDR-/XDR-Tuberkulose in Deutschland, Presentation at „Tagung zum Welttuberkulosetag, RKI, Berlin, accessed from:https://www.rki.de/DE/Content/InfAZ/T/Tuberkulose/WTBTag2014/Vortrag_04.pdf?__blob=publicationFile

ECDC (2018) Tuberculosis surveillance and monitoring in Europe 2018 – 2016 data, Stockholm, European Centre for Disease Prevention and Control

Fiebig, L., Hauer, B., Brodhun, B., Altmann, D., Haas, W. (2015) Tuberculosis in Germany: a declining trend coming to an end?, Eur Respir J (47), pp 667-670

Hillienhof, A. (2016) Infektionen; Mehr Tuberkulose-Fälle in Deutschland, Dtsch Arztebl International 113(12), p 522

Jacob, J.T., Mehta, A.K., Leonard, M.K. (2009). "Acute forms of tuberculosis in adults". The American Journal of Medicine. 122 (1): 12–7. doi:10.1016/j.amjmed.2008.09.018. PMID 19114163.

Kaufmann, S.H. and Schrager, L. (2016) Wir benötigen dringend eine neue Impfung, FAZ Wissen, accessed from: https://www.faz.net/aktuell/wissen/medizin-ernaehrung/wir-benoetigen-dringend-eine-neue-tuberkulose-impfung-14138766.html?printPagedArticle=true#void

Kerksiek, K. (2009) *Tuberkulose: Eine lange Geschichte mit ungewissem Ausgang*, InfectionResearch, accessed from:http://www.dzif.de/fileadmin/user_upload/Perspectives2009/September2009/TUBERK ULOSE_Eine_lange_Geschichte_22_09_2009.pdf

Kumar V, Abbas AK, Fausto N, Mitchell RN (2007). *Robbins Basic Pathology* (8th ed.). Saunders Elsevier. pp. 516–522. ISBN 978-1-4160-2973-1

Lawn, S.D., Zumla, A.I. (2011) "Tuberculosis". *Lancet.* **378** (9785): 57–72. doi:10.1016/S0140-6736(10)62173-3. PMID 21420161

Restrepo, B.I. (2007) "Convergence of the tuberculosis and diabetes epidemics: renewal of old acquaintances". *Clinical Infectious Diseases.* **45** (4): 436–8. doi:10.1086/519939. PMC 2900315. PMID 17638190

RKI (2013) Tuberkulose, RKI-Ratgeber, Berlin, Robert Koch Institut, accessed from: https://www.rki.de/DE/Content/Infekt/EpidBull/Merkblaetter/Ratgeber_Tuberkulose.html

RKI (2015) Thorax-Röntgenuntersuchungen bei Asylsuchenden gemäß § 36 Absatz 4 IfSG, Berlin, Robert Koch Institut, accessed from: https://www.rki.de/DE/Content/InfAZ/T/Tuberkulose/Tuberkulose_Roentgen-Untersuchungen_Asylsuchende.html

RKI (2015) Untersuchung auf Tuberkulose bei asylsuchenden Kindern und Jugendlichen < 15 Jahre, Berlin, Robert Koch Institut, accessed from: https://www.rki.de/DE/Content/InfAZ/T/Tuberkulose/Tuberkulose-Screening_Kinder.html

RKI (2018) Bericht zur Epidemiologie der Tuberkulose in Deutschland für 2017, Berlin, Robert Koch Institut, accessed from: https://www.rki.de/DE/Content/InfAZ/T/Tuberkulose/Download/TB2017.pdf?__blob=public ationFile

RKI (2018) Tuberkulose-Impfung in Deutschland?, Berlin, Robert Koch Institut, accessed from: https://www.rki.de/SharedDocs/FAQ/Impfen/Tuberkulose/FAQ01.html

Schaberg, T. (responsible) (2017) S2k-Leitlinie: Tuberkulose im Erwachsenenalter, Pneumologie 71, pp 325-397

Sundareshan, V. and Evans, M.E. (2009) Preventive Regimens for TB Disease (Treatment of Latent TB Infection), editors, Mainous III, A.G. and Pomeroy, C. (2009). *Management of antimicrobials in infectious diseases: impact of antibiotic resistance* (2nd rev. ed.). Totowa, N.J.: Humana Press. p. 74. ISBN 978-1-60327-238-4.

van Zyl Smit, R.N., Pai, M., Yew, W.W., Leung, C.C., Zumla, A., Bateman, E.D., Dheda, K. (2010). "Global lung health: the colliding epidemics of tuberculosis, tobacco smoking, HIV and COPD". *The European Respiratory Journal.* **35** (1): 27–33. doi:10.1183/09031936.00072909. PMC 5454527. PMID 20044459

World Health Organization. (2010)"Tuberculosis Fact sheet N°104", Geneva: World Health Organization

WHO (2014) Towards TB Elimination: An Action Framework for Low-Incidence Countries, Geneva, World Health Organization, accessed from: http://apps.who.int/iris/bitstream/handle/10665/132231/9789241507707_eng.pdf;jsessionid=6 64B32238FDA85F8BDE48CE9E7B8934C?sequence=1

WHO (2016) Global Tuberculosis Report 2016, Geneva: World Health Organization; p 27

WHO (2018) The Lancet Commission on Tuberculosis: building a tuberculosis-free world, Geneva: World Health Organization, accessed from: https://www.who.int/news-room/commentaries/detail/the-lancet-commission-on-tuberculosis-building-a-tuberculosis-free-world

WHO (2018) What is multidrug-resistant tuberculosis (MDR-TB) and how do we control it?, Geneva: World Health Organization accessed from: https://www.who.int/features/qa/79/en/

WHO (2018) Global Tuberculosis Report 2018, Geneva: World Health Organization; Licence: CC BY-NC-SA 3.0 IGO, p 43

Picture

Figures

Word Count

Introduction	414
Tuberculosis and ist Nature of Threat	1772
Response oft he Government	613
Conclusion	522
	3321

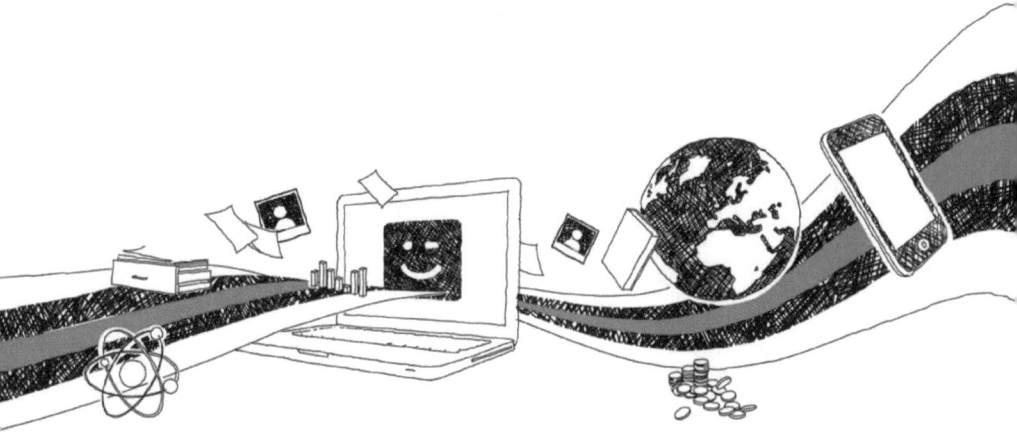
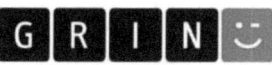